MULTIPLE SCLEROSIS (MS) DIET PLAN

Purposeful Diet For Brain And Spinal Health. Recipes Cookbook On Knowledge To Live Well, Manage, Strive And Reverse Neurological Disorders

DR. CHARLSE BLESSING

DISCLAIMER

The information in this book is meant solely for educational reasons. This book's contents are not meant to be used in place of expert medical advice, diagnosis, or treatment. Any decisions you make about your health must be discussed with a licensed healthcare provider.

Every effort has been made by the author to guarantee that the material in this book is correct and current as of the date of publication. Still, since medical knowledge advances rapidly, new studies might be conducted that change our understanding this illness and how best to manage it with food.

This book may contains references to and mentions of various people, things, websites, organizations, and other entities that the author does not support, advocate, or have any association with. There is no implied sponsorship or collaboration; all references and remarks are made only for informational purposes.

In order to address their individual health concerns, readers are advised to independently verify any information contained in this book and to consult with healthcare specialists. Any negative effects arising from the use or implementation of the material in this book, whether direct or indirect, are not the responsibility of the author or the publisher.

The dietary suggestions and counsel provided in this book are broad in scope and might not be appropriate for every individual. Readers are recommended to seek tailored counsel from trained healthcare specialists as individual health problems and demands differ.

The reader accepts the conditions of this disclaimer by reading this book.

FACTS ABOUT THIS BOOK

This book "Multiple Sclerosis (MS) Diet Plan" is one of the most important resources for anyone attempting to navigate the difficulties of life with multiple sclerosis (MS). This book discusses the critical relationship between nutrition and managing multiple sclerosis (MS) using an organized and enlightening style, highlighting the important role nutrition plays in symptom mitigation and enhancing general health.

This book's first sections give readers a comprehensive overview of multiple sclerosis by going over its definition, kinds, causes, and risk factors. By exploring the relationship between nutrition and MS symptoms, this book sheds light on how particular dietary choices can influence the progression of the disease, making a strong case for the adoption of a carefully curated MS diet plan. This basic knowledge serves as the basis for the subsequent investigation of the impact of diet on MS.

This book's emphasis on vital nutrients for managing multiple sclerosis is one of its main advantages. Through an exposition of the vitamins, minerals, antioxidants, and omega-3 fatty acids that are essential for people with multiple sclerosis, this book provides readers with the necessary information to make educated dietary choices. The list of certain items to eat and stay away from further helps readers create a balanced, customized MS diet.

A lot of attention is also given to the practical aspects of meal planning, including how to create balanced meals, how to use sample meal plans, and how crucial it is to modify a diet to suit each person's needs. Additionally, this book discusses particular issues that MS patients should be aware of, such as how to manage fatigue through diet, deal with weight issues, and comprehend how diet and medication may interact.

This book's comprehensive approach incorporates the synergy between exercise and nutrition, going beyond diet alone. This book emphasizes the value of a comprehensive wellness plan by detailing the advantages of exercise for MS patients and providing advice on modifying exercise to suit individual capacities.

Throughout this book, adopting new lifestyles is a major theme. It covers topics like stress reduction strategies, the effect of good sleep on MS, and striking a delicate balance between job, social life, and self-care. This book's dedication to enabling people on their MS journey is further demonstrated by the inclusion of long-term strategy, progress tracking, and professional support for maintaining the MS diet plan.

To sum up, the "Multiple Sclerosis (MS) Diet Plan" is an invaluable tool that provides a plethora of knowledge and helpful direction to people with MS who want to improve their quality of life by making thoughtful food selections and lifestyle changes.

CHAPTER ONE

OVERVIEW
A Synopsis Of Multiple Sclerosis

A chronic autoimmune disease that affects the brain and spinal cord, multiple sclerosis affects the central nervous system. It is typified by the immune system inadvertently targeting the myelin sheath that protects nerve fibers, causing communication breakdowns between the brain and the body as a whole. The symptoms of multiple sclerosis (MS) can vary greatly and include weakening in the muscles, numbness or tingling, fatigue, trouble walking, and issues with balance and coordination.

Recognizing the unexpected nature of MS is essential to comprehending its complexity. The condition's severity varies from person to person, and the symptoms may come and go. Although there is no known cure for multiple sclerosis (MS), there are several therapy modalities that attempt to control symptoms, impede the disease's advancement, and enhance the quality of life for those who have MS.

How Food Affects MS Management

The management of Multiple Sclerosis is heavily influenced by nutrition, and a new study indicates that specific dietary patterns may have an impact on the disease's severity and course. Although food cannot treat MS on its own, it can improve general health and possibly lessen certain symptoms. An important consideration is how diet affects inflammation, which is assumed to be a factor in the onset and course of MS.

Anti-inflammatory diets, like those high in antioxidants, plant-based foods, and omega-3 fatty acids, may help control MS symptoms. Walnuts, flaxseeds, and seafood are rich sources of omega-3 fatty acids, which have anti-inflammatory qualities that may help lessen inflammation in the central nervous system. Fruits and vegetables are rich in antioxidants, which can counteract free radicals and save nerve cells from harm.

Furthermore, because low levels of vitamin D are linked to an increased risk of developing MS, the vitamin has drawn attention in the context of managing the condition.

Vitamin D is commonly obtained from sun exposure, fortified foods, and supplements; keeping levels adequate may help reduce the symptoms of multiple sclerosis.

The objective and extent of the MS Diet Plan

An MS diet plan aims to maximize nutrition to maintain general health and possibly reduce some of the symptoms related to MS. The range includes a thorough approach to food selection, emphasizing items that may have a favorable effect on immunological response, inflammation, and general health.

A balanced and varied nutrient intake is usually emphasized by the MS Diet Plan, with a focus on whole foods. The main components of the diet include fruits, vegetables, whole grains, lean proteins, and healthy fats. Processed foods, which are heavy in carbohydrates and saturated fats, are often avoided since they might worsen general health and cause inflammation.

In addition, the MS Diet Plan could entail keeping an eye on particular nutrients, such as vitamin D, and thinking about supplements if needed. Customized eating plans consider the distinct requirements and inclinations of every individual suffering from multiple sclerosis, acknowledging that universal methods might not be appropriate.

In summary, the MS Diet Plan is a comprehensive strategy that supplements conventional medical treatments for the management of multiple sclerosis.

CHAPTER TWO

COMPREHENDING MULTIPLE SCLEROSIS
Types and Definitions of Multiple Sclerosis:

The autoimmune disease known as multiple sclerosis (MS) is a chronic, erratic condition that mostly affects the brain and spinal cord. Myelin, the covering that protects nerve fibers, is mistakenly attacked by the immune system in multiple sclerosis (MS), causing inflammation and damage. To enable efficient and seamless communication between nerve cells, myelin is essential. Numerous neurological symptoms arise from abnormalities in transmission caused by myelin breakdown.

There are various forms of MS, and each has special traits of its own. Relapsing-remitting MS

(RRMS) is the most prevalent type, marked by intervals of symptom flare-ups interspersed with intervals of either full or partial recovery. After an initial episode of RRMS, secondary progressive MS (SPMS) usually develops, with symptoms progressively getting worse over time without any noticeable relapses. Less often occurring primary progressive MS (PPMS) is characterized by a continuous progression of symptoms without noticeable relapses or remissions. A rare subtype of multiple sclerosis known as progressive-relapsing MS (PRMS) is typified by a disease history that worsens gradually with sporadic relapses.

Comprehending the distinct varieties of multiple sclerosis is vital to customize therapy strategies and actions to target the unique requirements and obstacles linked to each subtype.

Reasons and Danger Factors:

Although the precise etiology of multiple sclerosis is still unknown, it is thought to be the result of a confluence of environmental and genetic variables. Although possessing certain genetic components does not ensure the onset of MS, some genetic variances are linked to an elevated risk of the illness.

Smoking, poor vitamin D levels, and exposure to specific diseases are examples of environmental factors that have been connected to an increased risk of MS.

There is a big function for the immune system in MS. Immune cells misinterpret the myelin sheath in MS patients, resulting in inflammation and nerve damage. It is believed that environmental stimuli and genetic predisposition both have an impact on this aberrant immune response.

Gender (women are more susceptible than men), age (MS is commonly diagnosed between 20 and 50 years old), family history of MS, specific infections, and geographic location (MS is more common in temperate regions) are some of the risk factors that can raise the possibility of getting MS.

Signs and Development:

Individual differences exist in the symptoms of multiple sclerosis, contingent upon the site and degree of nerve injury. Fatigue, trouble walking, tingling or numbness, weak muscles, issues with coordination, and eyesight impairments are typical symptoms. The way symptoms develop is not always predictable; some people may go through periods of stability, while others may see a reduction in function happen more quickly.

MS frequently manifests as exacerbations, or relapses, in which existing symptoms get worse or new ones appear. Periods of remission, in which symptoms either totally or partially improve, usually follow this. Disabilities may progressively accumulate over time, particularly in progressive types of MS.

MS can have a significant negative influence on mobility, cognitive function, and emotional health in day-to-day living. The unpredictable and fluctuating nature of MS symptoms makes treatment difficult and necessitates a multidisciplinary strategy that may involve physical therapy, medication, and lifestyle changes. For MS patients to maximize their quality of life and address the disease's dynamic nature, regular monitoring and plan modifications are crucial.

CHAPTER THREE

DIETARY INFLUENCE ON MULTIPLE SCLEROSIS
Relationship Between MS and Diet:

Research and interest in the connection between nutrition and multiple sclerosis (MS) have grown. Although there is no cure or direct treatment for multiple sclerosis (MS), nutrition has a big influence on how successfully people with the disease manage their symptoms and live their lives. In multiple sclerosis (MS), the immune system targets the sheath that surrounds nerve fibers, causing interference in brain-to-body communication. According to newly available research, specific dietary components may have an impact on inflammation and the immune system, two processes that are critical to the onset and course of multiple sclerosis.

The impact of inflammation is a crucial component of the diet-MS relationship. Certain diets have been linked to increased inflammation in the body, especially those that are heavy in sugar and saturated fats. Increased inflammation in the context of MS may worsen symptoms and may hasten the course of the illness. Conversely, a diet high in fruits, vegetables, and omega-3 fatty acids that reduce inflammation may also have protective benefits.

In addition, MS research has focused more on the gut-brain axis, a two-way communication pathway between the central nervous system and the gastrointestinal tract. Dietary factors can modify immunological responses and affect neuroinflammation by altering the gut flora. This complex interaction highlights the value of managing multiple sclerosis (MS) holistically, as dietary decisions affect the gut environment in addition to the immune system.

The Impact of Nutrition on Symptoms:

A person's diet has a significant impact on the symptoms they experience. Because MS symptoms can vary greatly, from fatigue and cognitive decline to motor dysfunction, it is important to have a sophisticated grasp of how dietary decisions might affect the disease. For example, energy levels and cognitive function—both of which are frequently impacted by MS—have been related to specific nutrients.

One common MS symptom that can be impacted by dietary changes is fatigue. For example, iron deficiency can exacerbate fatigue, and people with MS may be more vulnerable to nutritional deficiencies as a result of medication side effects or malabsorption. Maintaining sufficient nutrient intake, such as iron, B12 and D vitamins, and omega-3 fatty acids, can play a critical role in addressing fatigue and enhancing general energy levels.

Another area where diet is critical in MS is cognitive performance. The health of the brain has been linked to omega-3 fatty acids, which are found in fatty fish and some seeds. Antioxidants found in fruits and vegetables may also have neuroprotective properties. Since MS patients frequently struggle with cognitive impairment, including these nutrients in the diet is essential to promoting cognitive health.

The Value of an All-Inclusive MS Diet Plan

A comprehensive MS diet plan adopts a holistic approach to enhance general health and well-being, going beyond individual food recommendations. Due to the intricacy of multiple sclerosis and the wide range of symptoms it might cause, a comprehensive approach that takes into account both the individual nutrients and the overall dietary pattern is required.

A diverse range of nutrient-dense foods, including fruits, vegetables, whole grains, lean meats, and healthy fats, are usually part of a well-rounded MS diet plan. These foods contribute to overall nutritional balance by offering important vitamins, minerals, antioxidants, and fiber. Additionally, maintaining a healthy weight is important for people with MS since being overweight can worsen certain symptoms and limit mobility. A balanced diet can help with this.

A key element of an MS diet plan is water, in addition to particular nutrients. Maintaining adequate hydration is crucial for preserving optimal body functioning and can help with symptom management, especially when it comes to easing fatigue and problems with the bladder.

Additionally, a thorough MS nutrition plan considers personal preferences and differences. It acknowledges the significance of long-term, sustainable dietary modifications that people can stick to. Working together with medical specialists, such as registered dietitians, guarantees that the meal plan takes into account any potential nutrient deficiencies and is in line with each person's unique health demands.

In summary, a comprehensive and customized approach to diet is critical to the management of multiple sclerosis (MS). Through comprehension of the relationship between nutrition and MS, identification of how nutrition impacts symptoms, and execution of an all-inclusive meal plan, MS patients can take charge of their health and potentially modify the course of their disease.

CHAPTER FOUR

CRUCIAL ELEMENTS FOR MS ADMINISTRATION
Minerals and Vitamins MS Patients Need:

Since vitamins and minerals are important micronutrients that support overall health and nervous system function, their involvement in managing multiple sclerosis (MS) is critical. Vitamin D is especially crucial for MS patients. Studies indicate that low vitamin D levels are associated with a higher chance of acquiring multiple sclerosis (MS). Vitamin D also influences the immune system through immunomodulatory activities, which may lessen the intensity of MS symptoms.

Another crucial vitamin for MS patients is vitamin B12. Ensuring an adequate intake of vitamin B12 can contribute to the preservation of nerve function and potentially alleviate symptoms associated with multiple sclerosis (MS).

This vitamin is crucial for maintaining the health of nerve cells and supporting the production of myelin, the protective coating around nerves that are often damaged in individuals with MS.

Zinc and magnesium are two more minerals that help control MS symptoms. Because of its anti-inflammatory qualities and involvement in several cellular processes, magnesium may help to lessen inflammation associated with multiple sclerosis. Zinc, on the other hand, is important for managing multiple sclerosis since it enhances immunological function and may help control the immune response.

In summary, maintaining the general health and functioning of MS patients requires a diet high in vital vitamins and minerals, especially zinc, magnesium, vitamin B12, and vitamin D. These nutrients support immune system regulation, nerve health maintenance, and possibly even the lowering of MS-related inflammation.

<u>Vitamins and Their Function:</u>

Due to their ability to counteract oxidative stress, which is a process linked to the advancement of multiple sclerosis, antioxidants are essential for managing the condition. An imbalance between the body's antioxidants and free radicals causes oxidative stress, which damages cells. Antioxidants are essential for MS patients since they frequently have elevated oxidative stress.

Strong antioxidants like vitamins C and E can assist in scavenging free radicals, therefore preventing damage to nerve cells and myelin. Furthermore, foods high in beta-carotene, like sweet potatoes and carrots, offer an additional layer of antioxidant defense. Together, these antioxidants combat the oxidative stress that aids in the development of multiple sclerosis.

Because fruits and vegetables are rich in antioxidants, MS patients must include a wide range of fruits and vegetables in their diet. Anthocyanins, which are substances with strong antioxidant qualities, are abundant in berries in particular. These antioxidants may have anti-inflammatory properties in addition to their ability to fight oxidative stress, making them advantageous for people with multiple sclerosis.

In summary, people with MS must eat a diet high in antioxidants to reduce oxidative stress and its harmful effects on nerve cells. MS sufferers can improve their body's ability to combat the oxidative damage linked to the condition by including a variety of fruits, vegetables, and sources of vitamins C and E.

MS and Omega-3 Fatty Acids:

Omega-3 fatty acids—found in walnuts, flaxseeds, and fatty fish—particularly eicosapentaenoic acid (EPA) and docosahexaenoic acid (DHA)—have drawn interest due to their possible advantages in the treatment of multiple sclerosis. Since inflammation is a major aspect of MS, these fatty acids are well known for their anti-inflammatory qualities, which can be very helpful for those who have the condition.

According to research, omega-3 fatty acids may be able to lessen inflammation in the central nervous system and regulate the immune system. The anti-inflammatory impact of omega-3 fatty acids may help to preserve myelin, the protective sheath around nerves that is frequently damaged in MS patients and may also help to reduce symptoms and halt the disease's course.

For MS patients, including omega-3 fatty acid sources in their diet—such as walnuts, flaxseeds, and fatty fish like salmon, mackerel, and sardines—can be helpful. These foods offer a natural, all-encompassing method of reducing inflammation and promoting general neurological health in addition to being a source of vital nutrients.

In conclusion, because of their anti-inflammatory properties and capacity to maintain nerve health, omega-3 fatty acids are essential for managing multiple sclerosis. Including EPA and DHA-rich foods in the diet can be a beneficial part of an all-encompassing strategy for maintaining MS patients.

CHAPTER FIVE

ITEMS TO ADD TO YOUR MS DIET
Produce and Fruits:

Including a wide range of fruits and vegetables in a Multiple Sclerosis (MS) diet plan is essential for improving general health and controlling the autoimmune disease's symptoms. These nutrient-dense foods include vital vitamins, minerals, and antioxidants that are important for immune system support and inflammation reduction—two critical components of controlling multiple sclerosis.

Berries, leafy greens, citrus fruits, and colorful veggies are just a few examples of fruits and vegetables that are high in vitamins like C, which have antioxidant qualities that help fight oxidative stress. Consequently, antioxidants aid in shielding the body's cells from the harm that free radicals can do, which in turn can exacerbate inflammation. Furthermore, fruits and vegetables' high fiber content supports a healthy digestive tract and may help with constipation, a typical problem for people with multiple sclerosis.

Moreover, including fruits and vegetables in a diet for MS patients may aid with weight control, which is another important part of the disease. Those who manage their weight correctly can benefit from improved mobility and general well-being as they cope with the difficulties this condition presents.

Fiber and Whole Grains:

Whole grains and fiber are crucial components of an MS diet plan because they improve digestive health and provide a steady supply of energy, among other benefits. Complex carbohydrates, which are abundant in whole grains like brown rice, quinoa, oats, and whole wheat, are an important source of energy for people with MS, who may find that fatigue is a common symptom.

Fiber, which is abundant in whole grains, helps to keep the bowels regular and prevents constipation, which is a common issue for people with multiple sclerosis. Additionally, a diet rich in fiber promotes satiety, which helps to manage weight and may lower the risk of complications related to obesity.

Since whole grains frequently contain vital vitamins and minerals including B vitamins, magnesium, and zinc, which are critical for nerve function and general well-being, the nutritional profile of whole grains is especially important for people with MS. People with MS can maximize their nutritional benefits and minimize potential inflammatory triggers by selecting whole grains versus refined grains.

Trim Proteins:

An MS diet plan must include lean proteins since they provide important amino acids needed for muscle health, repair, and overall body function. Lean protein sources including chicken, fish, tofu, lentils, and low-fat dairy products can help preserve muscle mass and strength, which helps address one of the issues that people with MS confront.

Consuming protein is especially important for those with MS since it helps with immune system support and tissue healing. Furthermore, eating meals high in protein makes you feel fuller for longer, which helps you control your weight and may lower your chance of developing issues from obesity.

Lean proteins can be a source of omega-3 fatty acids, which have anti-inflammatory qualities, in addition to their function in maintaining muscle health. For people with MS, eating fish high in omega-3s, like mackerel or salmon, may be helpful since it may help control inflammation and possibly lessen some of the symptoms of the disease.

Good Fats:

An MS diet plan must include healthy fats because they have several advantages for both overall health and particular MS symptoms. Nuts, seeds, avocados, and olive oil are good sources of monounsaturated and polyunsaturated fats that support heart health and may have anti-inflammatory properties.

Omega-3 fatty acids are particularly significant for people with MS since they have been linked to a reduction in inflammation and may help manage symptoms like fatigue and cognitive dysfunction. These fats can be found in fatty fish like salmon, flaxseeds, and walnuts.

Furthermore, eating healthy fats in the diet aids in the absorption of vitamins that are soluble in fat, such as vitamin D. Since vitamin D levels are frequently lower in MS patients, it is essential to ensure appropriate intake of good fats for the health of your bones and immune system as a whole.

While healthy fats have many advantages, moderation is essential. Optimizing the advantages of a diet rich in healthy fats for people with MS requires maintaining a balanced ratio of different types of fats and avoiding excessive amounts of trans and saturated fats.

CHAPTER SIX

FOODS TO AVOID IN AN MS DIET
Possible Triggers and Aggravators:

Understanding potential triggers and aggravators that may aggravate MS symptoms is essential to developing a successful Multiple Sclerosis (MS) diet plan. Common triggers include dairy products, gluten, and nightshade vegetables. Certain foods may contribute to oxidative stress, inflammation, and immune system dysregulation—all of which are variables related to the progression of MS. Proteins included in dairy products can provoke an immunological reaction in certain people, which could exacerbate MS symptoms. Solanine, a chemical found in nightshade vegetables like tomatoes, eggplants, and peppers, may contribute to inflammation and may worsen MS symptoms in susceptible individuals. Gluten, which is found in wheat and other grains, is known to cause inflammation in some people and may have a similar effect on those with MS. One of the most important steps in using dietary interventions to manage MS is recognizing and removing these triggers.

Processed Foods and Additives:

People with MS should be very careful about consuming processed foods and the additives that go along with them because they are known to cause several health problems. Processed meals frequently have high sodium, bad fats, and artificial additives, all of which can cause oxidative stress and inflammation. Artificial colors, flavors, and preservatives are among the additives that may upset the immune system's delicate balance and hasten the course of MS. Additionally, processed foods are frequently devoid of vital nutrients, which can result in nutritional deficits that further impair the body's capacity to control the illness. A diet high in fruits, vegetables, lean meats, and whole grains, or whole foods, can help manage MS symptoms and reduce inflammation while also providing the nutrients required for good health.

Sugar's Effect on MS:

An essential component of any MS diet plan is understanding the association between sugar and Multiple Sclerosis. Consuming a lot of sugar has been connected to oxidative stress, insulin resistance, and inflammation—all of which can make MS symptoms worse. A diet high in sugar may also have a deleterious effect on the gut microbiome, which may have an impact on the course of MS. Eating a lot of refined sugars and high-glycemic foods can cause blood sugar levels to spike and crash, which can exacerbate fatigue and other neurological symptoms linked to MS. Instead, a low-sugar or sugar-free diet that emphasizes natural sources of sweetness, such as fruits, and chooses complex carbohydrates can help stabilize blood sugar levels and lessen the inflammatory effects of sugar consumption. Comprehending the complex relationship between sugar and multiple sclerosis (MS) is crucial for those seeking to enhance their dietary habits and control the disease's effects on their general health.

CHAPTER SEVEN

THE VALUE OF STAYING HYDRATED
The Function of Water in MS Management

A chronic autoimmune illness affecting the central nervous system, multiple sclerosis (MS) causes a variety of neurological symptoms. Even though there isn't a treatment for multiple sclerosis, following a balanced diet can help control symptoms and enhance general health. Maintaining adequate hydration is essential to a successful MS diet plan because water is essential for many physiological processes.

Water is vital for good health, but it's even more important for people with multiple sclerosis (MS). For starters, staying well-hydrated aids in the management of typical MS symptoms like fatigue.

Due to the increased energy demands on their bodies, MS sufferers frequently experience weariness; further exacerbation of this condition can occur from dehydration. People with multiple sclerosis may be able to reduce fatigue and improve their day-to-day functionality by drinking enough water.

Furthermore, water is essential for maintaining cognitive function, which is critical for MS patients in particular as they may have cognitive impairment.

Concentration, memory, and general cognitive function have all been related to dehydration. MS sufferers may be able to lessen these cognitive difficulties and preserve a better quality of life by making sure they are drinking enough water.

Furthermore, maintaining adequate hydrated is essential for assisting the body's natural detoxifying processes. Free radicals and toxins are produced as a result of immune system dysregulation and inflammation in multiple sclerosis.

Drinking enough water helps the kidneys remove these poisons, which improves internal health and may lessen the intensity of MS symptoms.

It's crucial to remember that maintaining proper hydration has benefits beyond symptom alleviation for MS patients. According to some research, preserving adequate amounts of hydration may help slow the disease's course.

Although further investigation is necessary to completely comprehend this connection, the possible advantages render hydration an essential element of an MS eating regimen.

Tips for Hydration for MS Patients:

Effective hydration techniques must be a regular part of life for people with MS to maintain general health and control symptoms. A few hydration suggestions catered to the unique requirements of MS patients are as follows:

1. Regular Water Intake: It's important to create a schedule for your regular water intake. This is drinking smaller amounts of water throughout the day as opposed to a huge one at once. This method lessens the chance of dehydration by helping to maintain water levels more steadily.

2. Monitoring Fluid consumption: It's crucial to keep an eye on your total fluid consumption in addition to water. Although the main source of hydration is water, hydrating foods and drinks like fruits, vegetables, and herbal teas can also help maintain a balanced fluid intake.

3. Adapting to Individual Needs: Different people experience MS symptoms and the disease's effects differently. For this reason, MS sufferers must modify their hydration intake according to their particular requirements. Hydration needs can be impacted by several variables, including the weather, degree of physical activity, and medications.

4. Electrolyte Balance: Individuals with Multiple Sclerosis (MS) should be mindful of their electrolyte balance, particularly if they are taking medication or exhibiting symptoms that could impact their electrolyte levels. Including foods and beverages high in electrolytes can support the maintenance of a balanced diet.

5. Steer Clear of Dehydrating chemicals: Alcohol and caffeine are two examples of chemicals that might cause dehydration. Patients with multiple sclerosis should be careful about the substances they take in and, if they do, balance them with more water.

To sum up, keeping yourself hydrated is essential to controlling MS symptoms and enhancing your general health. People with MS can take proactive measures to support their health and possibly enhance their quality of life by learning the importance of water in managing their condition and putting customized hydration guidelines into practice.

SECTION EIGHT

MEAL PREPARATION FOR PEOPLE WITH MS
Creating a Multiple Sclerosis (MS) Diet Plan with Balanced Meals

For those with Multiple Sclerosis (MS), developing a balanced food plan is essential to controlling symptoms and enhancing general well-being. A well-balanced diet helps sustain energy levels, attends to certain nutritional requirements, and aids in keeping a healthy weight.

First and foremost, it's crucial to include a range of nutrient-dense foods. For long-term energy production, the macronutrients—fats, proteins, and carbohydrates—must be in balance. Complex carbohydrates can be found in whole grains like brown rice and quinoa, which can be used as the foundation of meals. Lean protein sources that support muscle health and regeneration include fish, poultry, tofu, and lentils.

Including a diverse range of fruits and vegetables also contributes important vitamins, minerals, and antioxidants. For example, berries, citrus fruits, and leafy greens are full of nutrients that boost immunity and lower inflammation—two things that are very important for people with multiple sclerosis.

Nuts, avocados, and olive oil are good sources of healthy fats that are essential for brain function. Fatty fish, such as salmon, are high in omega-3 fatty acids, which may also have anti-inflammatory properties and help maintain cognitive function.

Another essential component of creating balanced meals is portion control. For people with MS, it's critical to maintain a healthy weight because being overweight can make symptoms worse. Keeping an eye on portion sizes promotes weight control by assisting in the regulation of calorie intake.

Although it's sometimes forgotten, maintaining adequate hydration is vital for people with multiple sclerosis (MS). It supports digestion, preserves cognitive function, and helps regulate body temperature—particularly for those who are heat-sensitive.

To support general health and symptom management, creating balanced meals for an MS diet entails carefully combining nutrient-dense foods, sensible portion sizes, and attentive drinking.

Multiple Sclerosis (MS) Diet Sample Menus

Developing sample meal plans for people with Multiple Sclerosis (MS) entails adjusting nutrition to meet individual requirements while maintaining palatability and diversity. To properly manage symptoms, individuals experiencing dietary changes can benefit from using sample meal plans as a reference.

The start of a normal day's food plan could be a hearty breakfast, such as a bowl of oatmeal with berries and almonds on top. Soluble fiber from oats provides long-lasting energy, antioxidants from berries and protein, and healthy fats from nuts.

A vibrant salad topped with grilled chicken, cherry tomatoes, avocado, and lush greens can provide a variety of protein, vitamins, and minerals for lunch. A dressing made with olive oil adds beneficial fats.

Between meals, you can have a piece of fruit and a tiny bit of cheese or Greek yogurt paired with a handful of walnuts as a snack. These choices offer a good ratio of carbohydrates, healthy fats, and protein.

A choice of roasted veggies along with quinoa and grilled fish or tofu might make up dinner. With quinoa providing a full protein source and fish providing omega-3 fatty acids, this combination guarantees a varied nutrient profile.

When making sample meal plans, it's critical to take dietary limitations and personal preferences into account. It may be simpler for people to follow the MS diet plan if recipes are modified to accommodate different taste preferences.

Furthermore, using locally and seasonally available products for meals improves their nutritional content and freshness.

Adapting a Diet to a Person's Specific Requirements in MS

Although there are broad recommendations for a food plan for people with Multiple Sclerosis (MS), it's important to identify and take into account each person's needs and preferences. Adapting the diet to individual circumstances guarantees a more enduring and pleasurable method of nutrition-based MS symptom management.

First and foremost, it's critical to comprehend particular food sensitivities or allergies. Certain foods, such as dairy or gluten, may cause sensitivity in certain MS patients. Reducing or avoiding trigger foods can help manage symptoms and enhance general health.

It's crucial to adjust the diet to each person's unique energy requirements. Calorie needs are influenced by variables like age, sex, activity level, and metabolic rate. Tailoring nutritional ratios and portion sizes guarantees that people get the energy they need without consuming too many calories. Furthermore, it's critical to take comorbidities into account when modifying the MS diet. It's possible for people with MS to also have other medical disorders like diabetes or cardiovascular problems, which call for certain dietary restrictions. Personalized advice can be obtained by working with healthcare providers, such as dietitians.

Following the MS diet plan requires careful consideration of cultural and personal preferences. Developing a diet that suits individual preferences and cultural customs increases the chances of long-term success. This could entail creating appropriate substitutions that satisfy dietary needs or modifying classic dishes.

Finally, constant observation and modification are necessary. Variations in MS symptoms and general health necessitate regular evaluations of the dietary regimen. Dietary recommendations are kept in line with each person's needs and health state when there is regular communication with healthcare experts.

To sum up, tailoring the MS diet to each person's requirements requires a unique and adaptable strategy. It guarantees that the diet plan is not only successful but also long-term sustainable when variables like dietary sensitivities, energy needs, comorbidities, and personal preferences are acknowledged and taken into account.

CHAPITRE NINE

PARTICULAR ATTENTION TO MS PATIENTS
Using Nutrition to Manage Fatigue:

A typical symptom of multiple sclerosis (MS) is fatigue, which requires good management to enhance overall quality of life. For MS patients, using particular dietary techniques can be quite helpful in reducing fatigue. First of all, a diet high in foods that provide energy, including complex carbs, can support sustained energy levels during the day. Whole grains, fruits, and vegetables are foods that release energy gradually, avoiding blood sugar crashes and spikes, which can exacerbate weariness.

In addition, being properly hydrated is crucial to overcoming weariness. Fatigue is one of the MS symptoms that can be made worse by dehydration. MS patients should prioritize drinking enough water and, if necessary, include items high in water, such as fruits and vegetables, in their diet. It's also a good idea to stay away from excessive alcohol and caffeine use, as both might lead to dehydration.

Micronutrients are just as important in regulating fatigue as macronutrients. It is crucial to make sure you are getting enough vitamins and minerals, especially iron, vitamin D, and B-complex vitamins. These nutrients affect fatigue levels and are involved in the metabolism of energy. Although eating a balanced diet is the best way to get these nutrients, supplementing may be taken into consideration with medical advice.

Walnuts, flaxseeds, and fatty fish are rich sources of omega-3 fatty acids, which have anti-inflammatory qualities and may help MS patients feel less worn out and irritated. Including these foods in the diet can be a beneficial tactic. It is imperative, therefore, to speak with a healthcare professional to ascertain specific requirements and possible drug interactions.

Taking Care of Weight Issues:

Given that both weight increase and reduction can affect how the disease progresses, weight management is important for people with multiple sclerosis. Keeping a healthy weight can have a good impact on energy and mobility and is essential for general well-being.

Eating a diet rich in nutrients and well-balanced is essential for MS sufferers. Prioritizing complete meals, such as fruits, vegetables, lean meats, and whole grains, can supply vital nutrients and aid with weight regulation. Portion management is also necessary to avoid overindulging because MS-related mobility problems may make physical activity difficult.

When mobility is impacted by MS symptoms, a qualified dietitian can create a customized meal plan that takes into account all restrictions and meets nutritional needs. Regular exercise that is within each person's capabilities can also help with weight management and general health.

It's critical to be aware of the emotional variables that could affect eating patterns. Anxiety, which is prevalent in MS patients, can cause emotional eating or appetite loss. These emotional components of weight management can be addressed by putting stress management strategies into practice, asking for help from medical professionals support groups, or both.

Interactions between Medication and Nutrition:

Managing the interplay between medicine and food is essential for people with multiple sclerosis. To control concomitant diseases, alter the course of the disease, or relieve symptoms, MS patients frequently use a variety of drugs. It is crucial to comprehend the potential interactions between nutrition and certain medications to maximize therapeutic results.

Medication absorption and effectiveness may be impacted by certain foods. For example, certain drugs may need to be taken with or without food to improve absorption or lessen adverse effects. For instance, grapefruit and its juice may interfere with the liver's ability to process several drugs.

While meals high in calcium are usually good for bone health, some drugs, such as those containing bisphosphonates, may not absorb well when consumed in this way. Consequently, MS patients and their medical team must have open communication on their dietary practices and any supplements they may be taking.

Additionally, MS patients need to be aware of certain dietary deficits brought on by their drugs. For example, bone loss and calcium depletion might result from the usual prescription of corticosteroids for MS exacerbations. In these situations, consuming more calcium and vitamin D through food or thinking about taking supplements might be essential.

In summary, the relationship between nutrition, weight control, and drug interactions is a complicated but essential part of providing comprehensive treatment for people with multiple sclerosis. A comprehensive MS care strategy must include techniques for addressing tiredness through nutrition, appropriate weight management, and knowledge of how nutrition interacts with drugs. People with MS can optimize their nutrition to improve overall well-being and manage the problems associated with the disease by collaborating with healthcare specialists.

CHAPTER TEN

EXERCISE AND THE MS DIET'S SYNERGY
Exercise's Benefits for MS Patients

Exercise has a multitude of physical, mental, and emotional advantages, making it an essential part of managing Multiple Sclerosis (MS). First off, cardiovascular health, which is frequently impaired in MS patients, can be improved with regular exercise. It increases cardiovascular fitness overall, improves blood circulation, and lowers the risk of heart-related problems. Exercise also helps people maintain a healthy body weight, which is essential for those with MS to adequately manage their symptoms.

Regular physical activity has also been demonstrated to increase mobility and flexibility, which lessens the effects of MS-related muscle spasms and stiffness. Preventing secondary problems including joint contractures and muscle atrophy is crucial. Exercise is also essential for improving balance and coordination, which helps to address some of the frequent issues that people with MS encounter.

Exercise is important because it improves mental health by lowering the risk of despair and anxiety that are frequently linked to long-term diseases like multiple sclerosis. It also releases endorphins, which are the body's natural mood enhancers and enhance general quality of life. Exercise also has significant benefits for the brain; research indicates that it may assist MS patients in preserving their cognitive function and slowing down the deterioration of their cognitive abilities.

Exercise in the context of multiple sclerosis (MS) is not only about maintaining physical health; it also plays a major role in managing fatigue, which is a common symptom of MS. Despite the common belief that exercise makes fatigue worse, appropriate physical activity has been demonstrated to increase energy levels and reduce fatigue related to MS.

In conclusion, exercise has numerous advantages for MS patients including improved physical, mental, and emotional health. People with MS can improve their overall health, effectively manage their symptoms, and improve their quality of life by making regular exercise a part of their routine.

Customizing Exercise to Each Person's Capabilities:

Exercise regimens should be customized to each person's capabilities to maximize benefits and reduce hazards, as symptoms and abilities vary greatly amongst MS patients. Recognizing the range of capacities among the MS community and using a customized approach to exercise prescription are two important tenets.

The symptoms of MS patients frequently fluctuate, with intervals of worsening and remission. Exercise regimens must therefore be flexible in light of the disease's changing nature. Depending on the person's present functional level, the amount, kind, and intensity of exercise should be adjusted to make sure the selected activities suit the person's capabilities and objectives.

Additionally, it's critical to include a range of workouts that focus on various facets of fitness. This includes strengthening activities to improve muscle function, flexibility exercises to treat stiffness, aerobic workouts to improve cardiovascular health, and balance exercises to lower the risk of falls. A well-rounded workout program promotes overall functional improvement by accounting for the various needs of people with multiple sclerosis.

Exercise regimens should be tailored to account for temperature sensitivity, with options for indoor or water-based activities that reduce the risk of overheating and exacerbation of symptoms. Heat sensitivity is a common challenge for people with multiple sclerosis, so it is imperative to consider this.

To sum up, customizing exercises to each person's skills necessitates a flexible and tailored strategy. Exercise regimens can be tailored to each individual with MS to promote physical well-being while reducing the chance of worsening symptoms by taking into account their individual needs and capacities.

Formulating a Plan for Holistic Wellness:

For those with Multiple Sclerosis (MS), a holistic wellness strategy goes beyond diet and includes a whole-person approach that takes into account lifestyle variables, mental health, and exercise. Recognizing the interdependence of several facets of well-being, this strategy seeks to address them in concert for the best possible health results.

A comprehensive wellness plan must include exercise if it is to improve physical health and lessen the effects of MS symptoms. This entails adjusting exercise regimens to each person's capabilities, accounting for the disease's unpredictable character, and taking into account elements like heat sensitivity. Through the integration of several exercise regimens, such as aerobic, strength, flexibility, and balance training, people with multiple sclerosis (MS) can reap comprehensive advantages that surpass mere physical health.

A holistic wellness plan also has to address mental health. Anxiety and sadness can arise as a result of the emotional toll that chronic illnesses like MS take on a person's emotional health. By including counseling, mindfulness exercises, and stress management strategies in the wellness plan, people can be better equipped to handle the emotional difficulties brought on by multiple sclerosis.

In addition, lifestyle elements including social networks, diet, and sleep quality are crucial for general wellness. While fatigue, a typical symptom of multiple sclerosis, must be managed, getting enough sleep is essential. A balanced, nutrient-rich diet also promotes general health. For people with MS, social networks and a caring community can foster a positive outlook and improve their general quality of life.

To sum up, a comprehensive wellness plan for multiple sclerosis entails a multimodal strategy that takes into account behavioral, mental, and physical aspects. People with MS can maximize their overall well-being, effectively manage their symptoms, and lead happy lives despite the challenges presented by the condition by addressing these factors in concert.

CHAPTER ELEVEN

ACCEPTING LIFESTYLE MODIFICATIONS
Techniques for Stress Management:

It is well-recognized that stress can worsen the symptoms of Multiple Sclerosis (MS) and accelerate the illness's course. For this reason, people with MS must use effective stress management practices. Mindfulness meditation, for example, has demonstrated the potential to lower stress levels among MS patients. By adopting this approach, stressors are lessened, relaxation is encouraged, and attention is brought to the present moment. Deep breathing techniques and yoga can also be helpful since they help control the autonomic nervous system, which lowers stress.

Furthermore, it has been demonstrated that cognitive-behavioral therapy (CBT), which focuses on recognizing and altering unfavorable thought patterns and behaviors, can help people with chronic illnesses—including multiple sclerosis (MS)—manage stress.

In addition to offering emotional support, support groups and counseling enable people with multiple sclerosis (MS) to exchange experiences and stress-reduction techniques.

Including enjoyable and relaxing hobbies and pastimes is another essential component of stress management. People with MS can find a mental respite from the challenges of their condition by participating in therapeutic activities like art, music, or nature walks.

People need to identify the things that trigger their stress and customize their stress management strategies to fit their individual needs and preferences.

The Benefits of Good Sleep for MS Patients

Good sleep is essential for general health and well-being, and for people with multiple sclerosis (MS), it is even more important. MS patients frequently experience sleep abnormalities, which must be addressed to control symptoms and advance general health. Better sleep quality can be achieved by establishing a regular sleep schedule, making your bedroom cozy, and using relaxation techniques before bed.

Studies have indicated a reciprocal association between sleep and symptoms of multiple sclerosis. Excessive sleep can exacerbate symptoms of multiple sclerosis (MS), such as weariness, impaired cognitive function, and mood swings. However, MS's inflammatory nature can also affect how people sleep. For this reason, it becomes essential for people with MS to implement techniques to improve the quality of their sleep.

Better sleep can be facilitated by taking care of things like bladder control and temperature regulation, which are major concerns for people with multiple sclerosis. Better sleep hygiene can also be achieved by avoiding stimulants such as caffeine and electronics close to bedtime. Healthcare professionals may also investigate drugs or therapy designed to specifically address certain sleep issues in MS patients.

For those who are managing multiple sclerosis (MS), realizing the connection between sleep and the disease and making good sleep hygiene a priority can have a favorable influence on daily functioning, mood, and overall quality of life.

Juggling Social Life, Work, and Self-Care:

One of the most challenging but important aspects of living with multiple sclerosis (MS) is finding a balance between work, social life, and self-care. When it comes to employment, this may mean talking to employers about remote work choices, flexible work hours, or accommodations. For people with MS to be able to sustain a meaningful and long-lasting career, they must speak up for their demands at work.

It takes careful juggling to fit professional obligations, social obligations, and self-care into your schedule. Social connection can offer a sense of community and emotional support, both of which are essential for mental health. Nonetheless, to avoid burnout and an aggravation of MS symptoms, it's just as crucial to pay attention to one's health and emphasize self-care.

A variety of practices fall under the umbrella of self-care, such as consistent exercise, a healthy diet, and making time for hobbies and leisure. It's important to strike the correct balance between exercise and rest because pushing yourself too hard might exacerbate your symptoms and cause exhaustion. Making use of adaptive techniques and assistive technology can promote freedom and simplify daily duties.

In summary, managing the complex facets of living with multiple sclerosis necessitates a comprehensive strategy that takes into account the relationships between stress reduction, restful sleep, and striking a balance between employment, social obligations, and self-care. Tailored approaches, continuous dialogue with medical professionals, and a strong support system are crucial elements in adopting lifestyle modifications that enhance the quality of life for people with multiple sclerosis.

CHAPITRE TWELVE

MAINTAINING THE MS NUTRITION PLAN
Long-Term Success Methods

Following an MS diet plan requires putting into practice an effective long-term strategy. Creating enduring routines that comply with dietary guidelines is essential for controlling MS symptoms. It's critical to see the diet plan as a way of life rather than a short-term solution. A well-rounded and balanced approach to nutrition is ensured by incorporating a variety of nutrient-dense foods, such as fruits, vegetables, lean meats, and whole grains. This helps meet the dietary requirements unique to people with multiple sclerosis in addition to promoting general health.

Maintaining consistency is essential for long-term success. Dietary compliance can be maintained by establishing a schedule for meal planning, preparation, and mindful eating. Regular consumption of vital nutrients—such as vitamins, antioxidants, and omega-3 fatty acids—can have a beneficial effect on the inflammation and immune system related to multiple sclerosis. Gradual dietary modifications also facilitate easier adaptation and lessen the chance of feeling overwhelmed.

Stressing the value of staying hydrated is yet another essential long-term tactic. Maintaining adequate hydration promotes general health and helps reduce certain typical MS symptoms. Drinking enough water promotes healthy circulation, digestion, and overall body function. When adhering to an MS diet plan, people should make drinking water their priority and think about including hydrating items in their regular meals, like fruits and vegetables.

Incorporating consistent physical activity into the long-term plan also helps with MS symptom management and promotes general well-being. Exercise has been demonstrated to enhance muscle strength, balance, and mood—all of which are especially important for people with multiple sclerosis (MS). Customizing exercise regimens to a person's interests and abilities guarantees sustainability and enjoyment, which increases the likelihood that a person will follow the long-term plan.

Monitoring Development and Modifying the Plan

To determine whether the MS diet plan is effective and to make the required modifications, effective progress monitoring is necessary. Individuals can track their eating habits and detect patterns and potential triggers for MS symptoms by keeping a thorough food diary.

Reviewing this journal regularly sheds light on how particular diets affect managing symptoms and general well-being.

It's critical to check food intake in addition to keeping an eye on one's emotional and physical health. Keeping track of changes in mood, energy level, and symptom severity aids in determining how well the diet plan is working for the individual. It's critical to recognize that development might not be linear and that setbacks might serve as opportunities for improvement and learning.

A critical element of long-term effectiveness is tailoring the MS diet plan according to each person's response. Seeking advice and helpful insights from healthcare specialists, such as nutritionists or registered dietitians, might be beneficial. These experts can offer assistance in interpreting progress data, pointing out possible areas for development, and formulating tailored suggestions. The long-term durability of the diet plan is improved by its flexibility, which enables adjustments based on personal needs and preferences.

Seeking Expert Advice and Assistance

Starting an MS eating plan can be difficult, therefore getting expert advice is essential to making the most of this journey. Medical experts who specialize in MS, such as neurologists and registered dietitians, can offer personalized guidance based on a patient's health status, symptomatology, and dietary requirements.

Personalized food recommendations can be provided by a registered dietitian with MS-specific experience, who will consider individual symptoms and any medication interactions. They can assist people in developing a diet plan that is nutrient-dense, well-balanced, and respectful of cultural norms.

It is essential to schedule routine check-ups with medical specialists to track development and modify the MS diet plan as necessary. These check-ins offer a chance to talk about any difficulties, deal with issues, and get continuing assistance. Healthcare practitioners can also do evaluations to monitor alterations in cognitive and physical abilities, assisting people in comprehending how the diet plan affects their general health.

Establishing a support network is crucial for long-term success, in addition to expert advice. Making connections with people who have MS or are on a comparable eating plan fosters a sense of shared experiences and community. Online and off, support groups provide a forum for people to talk about their experiences, share strategies, and ask for help when they're struggling.

In conclusion, maintaining long-term results with an MS diet plan necessitates a multimodal strategy that combines ongoing progress monitoring, long-term tactics, and expert advice. Through nutritional treatments, people with MS can manage their problems and ultimately improve their overall quality of life by adopting a flexible and holistic approach.